Chronic Wasting Disease

A Comprehensive Guide to Understanding, Preventing, and Managing this Disease

Linda Harrell

All rights reserved. No part of this publication may be reproduced, distributed,or transmitted in any form or by any means, including photocopying, recording, or other electronic or mechanical methods, without the prior written permission of the publisher, except in the case of brief quotations embodied in critical reviews and certain other noncommercial uses permitted by copyright law.

Copyright © Linda Harrell, 2023.

Table of Content

Introduction
- Definition of Chronic Wasting Disease (CWD)
- Significance of CWD in Wildlife
- The Origin and Discovery of CWD

Chapter 1

Understanding CWD
- The Science Behind Prion Diseases
- Mechanism of CWD Transmission
- Species Affected by CWD

Chapter 2

Symptoms and Diagnosis
- Clinical Manifestations in Animals
- Techniques for Diagnosing CWD
- Challenges in Early Detection

Chapter 3

CWD and Human Health
- Current Understanding of CWD's Relationship to Human Health
- Potential Risks and Concerns
- Studies and Research on CWD Transmission to Humans

Chapter 4

Preventive Measures
- Guidelines for Hunters
- Safety Precautions in CWD-affected Areas

Chapter 5

Management and Control
- Challenges in Eradicating CWD
- Case Studies of CWD Management Programs
- International Efforts in CWD Control

Chapter 6

Economic and Ecological Impact
- Impact on Wildlife Populations
- Effects on Local Economies
- Long-term Ecological Consequences

Conclusion

Introduction

Chronic Wasting Disease (CWD) stands as a formidable challenge at the intersection of wildlife health, conservation, and human well-being. In this introductory chapter, we delve into the essential aspects that set the stage for a deeper understanding of CWD.

Definition of Chronic Wasting Disease (CWD)

At its core, CWD is a progressive, fatal neurodegenerative disorder affecting cervids—animals belonging to the deer family, including deer, elk, moose, caribou, and reindeer. Unlike traditional infections, CWD is not caused by bacteria or viruses but by prions—misfolded proteins that trigger a chain reaction, leading to the degeneration of brain and nervous system tissues. The term "chronic wasting" encapsulates the profound weight loss and deterioration observed in animals affected by this enigmatic disease.

Significance of CWD in Wildlife

CWD holds profound significance in the realm of wildlife. Its impact extends beyond individual animals to influence population dynamics, ecosystem health, and the delicate balance of nature. As we explore the implications of CWD on wildlife, we'll uncover how the disease disrupts natural behaviors, alters migration patterns, and poses challenges to the sustainability of various cervid species.

The Origin and Discovery of CWD

The inception of chronic wasting disease can be attributed to the keen observations of American wildlife veterinarian **Beth S. Williams**. In her pioneering work, Williams conducted post-mortem examinations on deer and elk afflicted by an enigmatic syndrome. Through her discerning analysis, she identified distinct brain lesions aligning with transmissible spongiform encephalopathy (TSE). Collaborating with neuropathologist Stuart Young in 1978, they co-authored the inaugural scientific paper officially labeling the ailment as chronic wasting disease and delineating its characteristics within the TSE spectrum.

The discovery of CWD raised critical questions about its transmission pathways, ecological consequences, and the intricate interplay between captive and wild populations. We explore the historical timeline of CWD, shedding light on the pivotal moments that shaped our awareness of this unique and concerning affliction.

As we embark on this exploration of CWD, the complexities of its nature and the far-reaching implications become apparent. This book aims to unravel the layers of this disease, offering readers a comprehensive guide to navigate the scientific, ecological, and societal dimensions of chronic wasting disease.

Chapter 1

Understanding CWD

Chronic Wasting Disease (CWD) presents a complex intersection of biology, pathology, and ecological dynamics. To comprehend the intricacies of CWD, we delve into the scientific underpinnings, exploring the science behind prion diseases, the specific mechanisms driving CWD transmission, and the diverse array of species impacted by this enigmatic affliction.

The Science Behind Prion Diseases

At the heart of CWD lies a unique class of infectious agents – prions. Unlike conventional pathogens such as viruses or bacteria, prions are misfolded proteins that possess the ability to induce similar misfolding in normal, healthy proteins. This aberrant conformation triggers a cascade effect, leading to the accumulation of insoluble protein aggregates, primarily in the brain and nervous system.

In the context of CWD, the prions responsible for the disease are elusive agents that defy traditional notions of infection. Their resilience to standard sterilization methods and resistance to typical decontamination procedures make prions a formidable challenge in disease management. Understanding the molecular intricacies of prions is pivotal in deciphering how CWD takes root and propagates within cervid populations.

Mechanism of CWD Transmission

CWD spreads through a variety of routes, primarily involving direct and indirect contact. Direct transmission occurs through the exchange of bodily fluids such as saliva, feces, blood, or urine between infected and susceptible individuals. Indirect transmission, on the other hand, involves exposure to environments contaminated with infectious prions, a factor that complicates disease control measures.

The ease with which CWD is transmitted poses a significant challenge for wildlife management. Infected individuals shed prions into the environment, creating hotspots of contamination. This environmental persistence contributes to the longevity of CWD, rendering eradication efforts exceedingly difficult.

As we unravel the transmission dynamics, it becomes evident that CWD is not confined solely to the individual animal level but operates within a broader ecological context, influencing interactions between cervid species and their environment.

Species Affected by CWD

CWD exhibits a broad host range, affecting various species within the cervid family. Deer, elk, moose, caribou, and reindeer all fall prey to this insidious disease. The susceptibility of multiple species raises concerns about the potential cascading effects on ecosystem health and biodiversity.

Understanding the spectrum of affected species is crucial for assessing the ecological impact of CWD. Different species may exhibit varying levels of susceptibility, influencing the disease's prevalence and spread. The intricate web of interactions within cervid populations further complicates the management and mitigation of CWD.

As we scrutinize the species affected by CWD, it becomes apparent that unraveling the ecological intricacies is paramount. The interconnectedness of wildlife species, coupled with the persistent nature of prions in the environment, underscores the urgency of a holistic approach to comprehend and combat this devastating disease.

In this chapter, we've laid the foundation for comprehending the fundamentals of CWD. From the enigmatic science of prions to the intricate web of transmission mechanisms and the diverse spectrum of affected species, the journey into the depths of chronic wasting disease is only beginning. As we navigate further, the challenges and complexities of CWD will unfold, demanding a concerted effort from scientists, wildlife managers, and society at large to address this pervasive threat to wildlife health and conservation.

Chapter 2

Symptoms and Diagnosis

Understanding Chronic Wasting Disease (CWD) requires a close examination of the clinical manifestations in affected animals, the techniques employed for diagnosis, and the inherent challenges in detecting this insidious ailment at its early stages.

Clinical Manifestations in Animals

CWD manifests in a range of symptoms that collectively contribute to the devastating impact on cervid populations. The disease's progression is insidious, often taking months or even years before noticeable clinical signs emerge. Clinical manifestations in animals include a combination of behavioral changes and physical deterioration.

One prominent sign is drastic weight loss, leading to a condition known as "wasting." Infected animals may exhibit lethargy, disorientation, and an overall decline in normal behaviors. As the disease advances, affected cervids often display abnormal behaviors such as repetitive walking patterns, excessive salivation, and a vacant or fixed stare. These observable symptoms collectively paint a poignant picture of the toll CWD takes on the neurological and physiological well-being of affected animals.

Techniques for Diagnosing CWD

Accurate and timely diagnosis of CWD is paramount for effective disease management. Various techniques are employed to detect the presence of CWD-associated prions in affected animals. Post-mortem examination of brain and lymphoid tissues remains the gold standard for definitive diagnosis.

Immunohistochemistry and immunoblotting are laboratory techniques that involve the detection of abnormal prion proteins in tissues. Additionally, techniques such as enzyme-linked immunosorbent assay (ELISA) and real-time quaking-induced conversion (RT-QuIC) provide alternative methods for detecting prions with varying degrees of sensitivity and specificity.

The development of ante-mortem diagnostic tools, allowing for the detection of CWD in live animals, has become an active area of research. Techniques such as tonsil biopsy, rectal biopsy, and blood tests aim to provide non-invasive options for diagnosing CWD without the need for euthanasia.

Challenges in Early Detection

Early detection of CWD poses significant challenges due to the prolonged incubation period and the subtlety of initial symptoms. Infected animals may appear healthy during the early stages of the disease, making it difficult to identify and isolate affected individuals within populations.

Moreover, the elusive nature of prions adds another layer of complexity to early detection efforts. Prions are notoriously resistant to standard decontamination methods, and their presence in the environment can persist for extended periods. This persistence complicates attempts to identify and mitigate disease hotspots.

The asymptomatic phase of CWD further exacerbates the challenge of early detection. By the time clinical signs become apparent, the disease may have already spread within cervid populations. This delayed recognition hampers proactive management strategies, emphasizing the need for improved surveillance and diagnostic tools.

In this chapter, we've explored the nuanced landscape of CWD symptoms and diagnosis. From the subtle yet impactful clinical manifestations in animals to the intricacies of diagnostic techniques and the formidable challenges in early detection, our understanding of CWD deepens. As we navigate the scientific terrain of this disease, the urgency of refining diagnostic methods and bolstering surveillance becomes increasingly evident, highlighting the critical role these elements play in the broader context of managing and mitigating the impact of chronic wasting disease.

Chapter 3

CWD and Human Health

The intersection of Chronic Wasting Disease (CWD) and human health introduces a complex landscape, raising questions about the potential risks and the current understanding of any link between CWD and human well-being. In this chapter, we delve into the evolving narrative surrounding CWD and its implications for those who share ecosystems with infected cervids.

Current Understanding of CWD's Relationship to Human Health

As of the latest scientific understanding, there is no conclusive evidence that CWD can infect humans. CWD belongs to the family of prion diseases, which includes notorious afflictions like Creutzfeldt-Jakob Disease (CJD) in humans and Bovine Spongiform Encephalopathy (BSE), commonly known as mad cow disease. While these diseases share the prion pathology, the specific strain of prions causing CWD appears distinct from those associated with human prion diseases.

However, it's essential to approach this understanding with caution, recognizing the inherent challenges in studying zoonotic potential—the ability of an animal disease to jump to humans. The complex nature of prions and the extended latency periods in human prion diseases underscore the need for ongoing research to definitively establish the risk, if any, of CWD transmission to humans.

Potential Risks and Concerns

Despite the lack of documented cases of CWD in humans, the scientific community remains vigilant due to the unpredictable nature of prion diseases. The potential risks arise from the shared environments between infected cervids and humans, particularly in regions where CWD is prevalent. Exposure pathways include the consumption of contaminated meat, handling infected animals, or exposure to environments contaminated with CWD prions.

Concerns escalate when considering the cumulative exposure over time, especially for communities reliant on cervid populations for sustenance or recreational activities like hunting. The importance of addressing these concerns lies not only in potential direct transmission but also in the economic and cultural impacts on societies intertwined with cervid ecosystems.

Studies and Research on CWD Transmission to Humans

Scientific exploration into the zoonotic potential of CWD has intensified in response to concerns and the inherent uncertainties surrounding prion diseases. Various studies have been conducted to investigate the transmissibility of CWD to non-human primates—a crucial step in understanding the potential risks to humans.

Results from some studies suggest that certain non-human primates, like macaques, can be infected with CWD under experimental conditions. These findings, while raising concerns, do not directly translate to human susceptibility, and caution is warranted in extrapolating these results to broader populations.

The World Health Organization (WHO) has emphasized the importance of preventing the entry of prions from all known prion diseases, including CWD, into the human food chain. This precautionary approach aligns with the principle of minimizing potential risks to human health.

In navigating the intricate landscape of CWD and human health, ongoing research is paramount. The scientific community's collective efforts seek not only to ascertain the zoonotic risk but also to establish comprehensive guidelines for mitigating potential exposure. As we continue to unravel the mysteries of prion diseases, collaboration between wildlife experts, public health officials, and the communities affected by CWD remains essential to ensuring the well-being of both wildlife and humans sharing these ecosystems.

Chapter 4

Preventive Measures

Preventing and managing Chronic Wasting Disease (CWD) demands a multifaceted approach that involves active participation from hunters, communities, and governmental bodies. In this chapter, we explore the preventive measures aimed at curtailing the spread of CWD and minimizing potential risks to both wildlife and human populations.

Guidelines for Hunters

Hunters play a crucial role in the prevention and surveillance of CWD. Implementing and adhering to specific guidelines can contribute significantly to minimizing the risk of CWD transmission.

1. **Surveillance and Testing:** Hunters are encouraged to submit harvested animals for CWD testing, particularly in regions where the disease is prevalent. This active surveillance not only aids in early detection but also provides valuable data for wildlife management.

2. **Avoiding Sick-Looking Animals**: Hunters are advised to exercise caution and avoid harvesting animals that exhibit unusual behavior or appear sick. Symptoms such as excessive salivation, emaciation, or erratic movements may indicate CWD infection.

3. **Safe Handling and Processing:** Implementing proper field-dressing and processing techniques is crucial. Wearing gloves, avoiding direct contact with potentially infected tissues, and using dedicated tools for processing game are recommended practices.

4. **Disposal of High-Risk Parts:** Certain parts of the harvested animal, such as the brain and spinal cord, carry a higher risk of prion

concentration. Proper disposal methods, such as burying or incinerating these parts, help minimize environmental contamination.

Safety Precautions in CWD-affected Areas

Communities residing in or near CWD-affected areas should be aware of safety precautions to reduce the risk of exposure.

1. Public Awareness: Educational campaigns and outreach efforts are vital to inform residents about CWD, its symptoms, and preventive measures. Knowledgeable communities are better equipped to take precautionary actions.

2. Avoiding Direct Contact: Residents and outdoor enthusiasts should avoid direct contact with wildlife, especially sick or dead animals. Alerting local authorities when encountering such situations enables timely response and intervention.

3. Environmental Decontamination: CWD prions persist in the environment, posing a risk to both animals and humans. Implementing measures such as thorough cleaning of tools, equipment, and clothing after outdoor activities helps mitigate the potential spread of prions.

As we navigate the landscape of preventive measures against CWD, it is evident that a collective and informed effort is crucial. The collaboration between hunters, communities, and governmental bodies forms the backbone of effective prevention and management strategies. By implementing these measures, we strive to strike a balance between wildlife conservation, human health, and the preservation of cherished cultural practices such as hunting. In the subsequent chapters, we will explore the economic and ecological impact of CWD, examine specific cases like the Yellowstone incident, and discuss the global spread of this challenging disease.

Chapter 5

Management and Control

Effectively managing and controlling Chronic Wasting Disease (CWD) poses significant challenges due to its complex nature and the elusive characteristics of prion diseases. In this chapter, we explore the hurdles in eradicating CWD, examine case studies of management programs, and delve into international efforts aimed at controlling the spread of this enigmatic affliction.

Challenges in Eradicating CWD

Eradicating CWD presents a formidable challenge, primarily due to the unique properties of prions and the complexities associated with wildlife populations.

1. **Environmental Persistence:** Prions responsible for CWD exhibit remarkable resilience in the environment. Traditional decontamination methods are often insufficient to eliminate these infectious agents from soil, vegetation, and water sources, contributing to the persistence and recurrence of the disease.

2. **Asymptomatic Carriers:** Infected animals can act as asymptomatic carriers, spreading the disease unknowingly. Identifying and culling infected individuals during the asymptomatic phase is challenging, as visible clinical signs only manifest in later stages of the disease.

3. **Lack of Vaccines and Treatments**: Unlike conventional infectious diseases, CWD lacks vaccines or treatments. The absence of targeted interventions makes it difficult to implement strategies for preventing the spread of the disease within wildlife populations.

4. **Population Density and Movement**: The dynamics of cervid populations, including high

population density and extensive movement, contribute to the rapid transmission of CWD. Containing the disease becomes intricate when considering the expansive territories these animals cover.

Case Studies of CWD Management Programs

Despite the challenges, various regions have implemented management programs to curb the spread of CWD. Case studies provide insights into the strategies employed and the outcomes achieved.

1. Wisconsin CWD Management Zone: Wisconsin has faced persistent challenges in managing CWD, particularly in the southern part of the state. The establishment of a CWD Management Zone involved intensified surveillance, targeted culling of infected deer, and restrictions on the movement of carcasses. The effectiveness of these measures is continually evaluated, providing valuable lessons for future management programs.

2. Colorado's Adaptive Management Approach: Colorado adopted an adaptive management strategy, incorporating ongoing research, collaboration with stakeholders, and adjustments to management practices based on evolving scientific understanding. This flexible approach recognizes the dynamic nature of CWD and seeks to adapt strategies accordingly.

3. Illinois' CWD Response: Illinois implemented a comprehensive CWD response plan, focusing on early detection, risk reduction, and public awareness. The plan involves surveillance, targeted culling in affected areas, and communication efforts to educate the public about CWD risks and preventive measures.

International Efforts in CWD Control

Recognizing the global impact of CWD, international collaboration has emerged to share knowledge, coordinate research, and develop unified strategies for control.

1. **The CWD Alliance:** The Chronic Wasting Disease Alliance in North America exemplifies collaborative efforts among wildlife agencies, researchers, and stakeholders. The alliance emphasizes information exchange, research coordination, and public outreach to enhance collective understanding and control measures.

2. **European CWD Initiative:** In Europe, where CWD has been reported in several countries, the European CWD Initiative fosters collaboration to address the challenges posed by the disease. The initiative focuses on harmonizing surveillance methods, sharing data, and developing region-specific strategies for CWD control.

3. **International Collaboration through OIE**: The World Organisation for Animal Health (OIE) plays a pivotal role in facilitating international collaboration on animal health issues. CWD has been recognized as a transmissible spongiform encephalopathy by the

OIE, emphasizing the need for global cooperation in monitoring and managing the disease.

In navigating the complexities of managing and controlling CWD, these case studies and international efforts underscore the importance of adaptive strategies, collaboration, and ongoing research. The lessons learned from diverse approaches contribute to a collective knowledge base, guiding future endeavors to mitigate the impact of CWD on wildlife populations and safeguard the health of ecosystems worldwide. In the upcoming chapters, we will delve into the economic and ecological impact of CWD, examine specific incidents such as the case in Yellowstone National Park, and explore the broader implications of this intricate and evolving challenge.

Chapter 6

Economic and Ecological Impact

Chronic Wasting Disease (CWD) extends its influence beyond individual animals, permeating wildlife populations, local economies, and the intricate web of ecological interactions. In this chapter, we explore the far-reaching economic and ecological consequences of CWD, shedding light on the profound ripple effect it casts across ecosystems.

Impact on Wildlife Populations

CWD's impact on wildlife populations is multifaceted, disrupting not only the health of individual animals but also the dynamics of entire ecosystems.

1. **Population Decline:** Infected animals face increased mortality, leading to potential declines

in cervid populations. This decline can reverberate through the food web, affecting predators that depend on cervids as a primary food source.

2. Altered Behavior and Social Structure: CWD-induced behavioral changes in affected animals can alter social dynamics within populations. Disorientation, reduced interaction, and altered migration patterns can disrupt established hierarchies and social structures.

3. Genetic Consequences: Selective pressure from CWD may impact the genetic diversity of cervid populations over time. The disease could potentially exert pressure on certain genetic traits, influencing the evolutionary trajectory of affected species.

Understanding these dynamics is crucial for wildlife managers seeking to assess and mitigate the cascading effects of CWD on biodiversity and ecological balance.

Effects on Local Economies

CWD's economic impact extends beyond wildlife, affecting local economies that rely on activities such as hunting, wildlife tourism, and associated industries.

1. Decline in Hunting Opportunities: Hunting is deeply intertwined with local economies, providing revenue through licenses, permits, and associated services. As CWD affects cervid populations, hunting opportunities may decline, impacting the income derived from these activities.

2. Reduced Tourism and Recreation: Areas with vibrant wildlife populations often attract tourists and outdoor enthusiasts. CWD can discourage visitation due to concerns about disease transmission, leading to diminished revenue for local businesses catering to tourism and recreation.

3. Economic Strain on Related Industries: Industries linked to hunting, such as taxidermy, meat processing, and equipment sales, may experience economic strain as CWD affects wildlife populations. The economic interconnectedness of these industries amplifies the impact across the local economic landscape.

The economic repercussions highlight the need for proactive management strategies that balance ecological preservation with the sustainable use of wildlife resources.

Long-term Ecological Consequences

The long-term ecological consequences of CWD are a subject of ongoing research and concern, with potential ramifications for biodiversity, ecosystem resilience, and overall ecological health.

1. Altered Plant-Herbivore Interactions: Changes in cervid populations can influence plant-herbivore interactions, impacting vegetation dynamics and plant community structure. This, in turn, may have cascading effects on other wildlife species dependent on specific vegetation types.

2. **Predator-Prey Dynamics**: The decline in cervid populations due to CWD can disrupt predator-prey dynamics. Predators that rely on cervids as a primary food source may face challenges, potentially leading to shifts in predator behavior or changes in local predator populations.

3. **Ecosystem Resilience**: CWD's impact on wildlife populations and ecological interactions could compromise ecosystem resilience. The ability of ecosystems to withstand and recover from disturbances may be compromised, posing challenges for maintaining balanced and healthy ecological systems.

The long-term ecological consequences of CWD underscore the importance of a holistic and adaptive approach to wildlife management, with an emphasis on preserving biodiversity and ecosystem function.

In conclusion, the economic and ecological impact of Chronic Wasting Disease transcends the boundaries of individual animals and ecosystems. Recognizing the interconnectedness of wildlife health, local economies, and ecological balance is essential for developing comprehensive strategies to address and mitigate the multifaceted challenges posed by CWD. In the subsequent chapters, we will delve into specific incidents such as the Yellowstone case, explore global perspectives on CWD, and examine the ongoing efforts to tackle this intricate and evolving issue.

Conclusion

As we conclude this journey through the intricate landscape of Chronic Wasting Disease (CWD), we find ourselves standing at the intersection of wildlife health, human impact, and ecological balance. The shadows cast by CWD extend far beyond the realm of individual animals, leaving an indelible mark on the intricate tapestry of nature.

In the depths of this exploration, we've uncovered the mysteries surrounding CWD, from its elusive prion pathology to the far-reaching consequences it imposes on wildlife populations, local economies, and the delicate dance of ecosystems. We've delved into the challenges of detection, the nuances of zoonotic potential, and the collective efforts required for prevention and control.

The tales of CWD unfold as cautionary whispers, urging us to tread carefully in the shared spaces between humans and wildlife.

From the silent forests to the bustling economies linked to hunting, every thread in this narrative is woven into the fabric of our interconnected world.

Yet, within the shadows, we find glimmers of resilience and hope. The dedication of scientists, wildlife managers, hunters, and communities in the face of this enigmatic adversary paints a canvas of collective determination. Case studies illuminate paths forward, demonstrating the adaptive strategies needed to navigate the ever-evolving challenges presented by CWD.

As stewards of our natural heritage, the responsibility to forge a sustainable coexistence falls upon us. The lessons learned from CWD beckon us to foster collaboration, embrace scientific inquiry, and reevaluate our relationship with the wild.

In the echoes of our exploration, let these insights guide our steps. May they inspire a future where the shadows of CWD yield to the light of understanding, resilience, and harmony. For in the heart of the wilderness, where challenges and mysteries converge, lies the promise of a world where humans and wildlife dance in sync, ensuring the vitality of our shared ecosystems for generations to come.

Made in United States
Orlando, FL
01 April 2024